T0250337

Power and Influence in the NHS

oceans without continents

Geoff Meads

Professor of Health Services Development
Health Management Group, City University, London

Foreword by

Peter Dickson

Professor Emeritus of Early Modern History
University of Oxford

Radcliffe Medical Press

© 1997 Geoff Meads

Radcliffe Medical Press Ltd
18 Marcham Road, Abingdon, Oxon OX14 1AA, UK

Radcliffe Medical Press, Inc.
141 Fifth Avenue, New York, NY 10010, USA

British Library Cataloguing in Publication Data

A catalogue record for this book is available from the British Library.

ISBN 1 85775 270 8

Library of Congress Cataloging-in-Publication Data is available

Typeset by Acorn Bookwork, Salisbury, Wilts
Printed and bound by Redwood Books, Trowbridge, Wilts

Contents

A new paradigm of public accountability
The spiritual dimension

Foreword

I was Geoff Meads's college tutor from 1970 to 1973. It is flattering a quarter of a century later to be asked by him to write the Foreword to his expert study, and to find that he is a professor too. His subject in this book, the modern NHS, seems to me every bit as complex and as difficult to grasp as the periods of history to which he refers.

He describes how the NHS has in the past decade moved away from central direction and planning structures towards local control centred on general practice fundholdings operating in an internal market. In the process, political conflict and power contests have been 'regionalized'. The underlying situation, which is outside the scope of this book, is that the allocation of scarce resources through a price-system responding to demand and supply, the normal commercial situation, is absent in health care, for whose consumers it is 'free at the point of sale'. Where there is no price constraint on demand, it becomes infinite. But since supply is not, demand is reined back by rationing, in the form of waiting lists and other devices. The internal market, the devolution of health care to local level, the importance of local initiatives, the variety of local practices, all of which Meads emphasizes, are, as I understand it, responses to this situation. They attempt to import enough of the discipline of the market into health care to make it adequately responsive to its consumers, while preventing escalation of its costs from forcing it into bankruptcy.

Together with social security and pensions, health care expenditure exerts a grip on the budgets of all western states similar to the grip which defence exerted during the Cold War. Meads hints in his interesting study that UK efforts to resolve this problem have proved superior to those of other European governments; and promise to do so in the future. The combination of effective administration and financial constraint which he describes is one of which the great Sir Robert Walpole, to whom he refers in Chapter 2, would have firmly approved.

Peter Dickson
Oxford
April 1997

Preface

Much of the content of the chapters that follow is devoted to identifying the changing interfaces of the NHS and the new opportunities for creativity that unexpected alliances, networks and coalitions can offer. This book owes its production to one such opportunity. The Director roles of an NHS Executive regional office and a university health management school are both new; archetypal spin offs of the contemporary NHS and clear evidence of the range of participants now joined in the UK health care system. Tony Laurance and Valerie Iles occupy these roles, in the NHS South and West Region and the Health Management Group of the City University respectively. Their joint ability to read the times and to supply the secondment opportunity through which this book has been created seemed far sighted in the spring of 1996. A year later I hope this foresight is still felt to have been worthwhile. This publication is by way of repayment to Tony and Valerie, to both of whom I owe a considerable debt.

I have enjoyed writing this book, and the refuge it represents after seven years spent in senior NHS management. It has been like learning to live again! The seven years mirror the seven chapters of the book which seeks to trace the development of the NHS, and to a lesser effect, the UK health care system, over this time. To describe and interpret this development a mixture of personal experiences and reflections, conceptual frameworks and parallels from the great periods of change of the past are deployed. To claim that the end result is multi-layered would be presumptuous. It is certainly, however, a curious mixture and for readers, as a minimum benefit, the figures distributed around the text provide a range of largely new change management methods and analytical techniques for use in practice.

I hope the book communicates. The format with its grand historic analogies, should not be taken too seriously; they have been fun to toy with as a vehicle for some simple and, I hope, true and striking assertions, albeit perhaps sometimes expressed too simplistically. I have learnt a great deal along the way. The experience has been a catharsis; making sense of what has gone before, finding a release to move on. I hope that at least for some readers it helps provide a similar step forward.

The book has also been a team effort. I am delighted to be able to acknowledge the crucial support I have received from Jane Harding for her sympathetic understanding and secretarial expertise; from Gillian Nineham and June Huntington whose editorial guidance and feedback respectively has been that of real friendship; and above all my gratitude goes to a partner whose tolerance and patience over the years has been *the* key. It is to her that I dedicate this book.

Geoff Meads
Winchester
April 1997

Abbreviations

AMGP Association of Managers in General Practice – nowadays the main national organization for Practice Managers which, over the past three years, has established itself as a counterpart to the Institute of Health Services Management.

BMJ British Medical Journal – the most widely read regular medical publication in the UK, and the most influential.

BUPA British United Provident Association – the leading private sector health care company in the UK.

CHC Community Health Council – consisting of local representatives responsible for ensuring local health services respond to the public interest.

CHS Community Health Services – include, for example, district nurses, health visitors, community hospitals and psychologists providing important specialist support to general practices.

DGH District General Hospital – since 1962 the main unit of NHS health care, usually providing for a population area of at least 150 000.

DHA District Health Authority – the pre-1996 title given to the 170 organizations responsible for purchasing secondary care services and promoting local health.

DoH   Department of Health – the central government department within which responsibility for the NHS is sited.

EL   Executive Letter – the usual method of communication used by the central management board of the NHS to convey its directions.

EU   European Union – based in Brussels and due to revise the very limited health component of its treaty in 1997/98.

FHSA   Family Health Services Authority – responsible for locally managing the nationally negotiated contracts of GPs, dentists, community pharmacists and opticians between 1990 and 1996, the year they were abolished.

FMR   Functions and Manpower Review – in 1993 led to a fundamental restructuring of management structures in the NHS including the abolition of RHAs and FHSAs in 1996.

GMC   General Medical Council – the supreme regulatory body for medical professionals.

GMS   General Medical Services – refers specifically to the services provided by GPs, subject to both national funding and negotiation, e.g. immunizations, consultations etc.

GMSC   General Medical Services Committee – comprises national GP representatives whose chief responsibility has been to negotiate annually the national terms of service for GPs.

GP   General Practitioner – according to all market research still the most appreciated professional in the contemporary NHS.

GPFH   General Practice Fundholding – the title given in 1990 to the subsequently much extended scheme whereby GPs acquire NHS budgets to purchase hospital and community health services.

HA   Health Authority – the new title given to the 101 organizations which replaced DHA's and FHSA's in April 1996, with responsibility for local NHS market oversight.

HCHS   Hospital and Community Health Services – prior to the 1997 legislation applied as the term for the financial allocations for all parts of the NHS, excluding primary care and prescribing.

HMG   Health Management Group, City University – academic base for the author and a leading provider of NHS management education.

HMSO   Her Majesty's Stationery Office – historically the main publisher of government documents.

HSG   Health Service Guidelines – a frequently used vehicle for central NHS communications usually in relation to service and clinical developments.

HSJ   Health Service Journal – the most popular and influential weekly publication for health care managers in the UK.

HSMC   Health Services Management Centre, Birmingham University – arguably the leading unit of its kind in the UK, led by Professor Chris Ham, with a considerable influence in national policy development.

KFOA   King's Fund Organizational Audit – a leading example of the new models of accreditation emerging in the NHS to which over 130 organizations subscribe; designed in London at the King's Fund Foundation.

LSE   London School of Economics – part of London University with a record of significant academic contributions to the NHS.

MENCAP   Royal Society for the Mentally Handicapped – the long established leading national charity for people with learning disabilities and their carers.

MIND   National Association for Mental Health – as for MENCAP but in relation to mental illness.

NAFP   National Association of Fundholding Practices – has over the past six years become an increasingly important mutual support and representative body for GPFHs, with a growing influence in national policy developments.

NHS   National Health Service – established in 1948 and now the largest public organization in Europe with over one million employees.

NHSE   National Health Service Executive – the title of the central headquarters Board of Directors for the whole NHS, sited at Quarry House in Leeds.

NHSME   National Health Service Management Executive – the pre-1993 title for the NHSE in England.

PCM   Primary Care Management – a leading monthly journal for managers in different areas of primary care.

PPG   Priorities and Planning Guidance – are issued by July of each year to set the annual strategic objectives and priorities for the whole NHS.

RAWP   Resource Allocation Working Party – gave its name, prior to 1990, to the NHS national funding formula for HCHS, largely based around hospital usage and catchment areas.

RCGP   Royal College of General Practitioners – the main professional body for GP's, although membership nationally is patchy.

RHA   Regional Health Authority – abolished in 1996 prior to which it was the chief strategic planning unit of the NHS, covering populations usually of between three and seven million.

SSI   Social Services Inspectorate – an arm of the Department of Health with a limited range of statutory oversight duties in respect of local social services departments.

UK   United Kingdom – the geographic territory for most of this book.

VFM   Value For Money – an audit criteria increasingly applied to NHS developments in relation to cost and clinical effectiveness.

'Inigo of Loyola caught a glimpse of the treasure within him by noticing the after-effects of his daydreams'*

To 'Tricia
with all my love

---

*From Gerard W Hughes (1994) *God of Surprises*. Darton, Longman and Todd, London, p 87.

1

Introduction:

manifesto

'Hereby it is manifest, that during the time men live without a
common power to keep them all in awe, they are in that
condition which is called Warre.'*

People are confused about the NHS. They know that its organization has changed, is changing, and they are not clear about where
in the future these changes are leading. This lack of clarity breeds
uncertainty which in turn too readily gives way to a pervasive sense
of insecurity. Given the scale of the NHS as a national institution
this affects the community at large and at all levels. It is a special
relationship. The NHS is a microcosm of society in the United
Kingdom; they create and re-create each other in their own images.

People are conscious of discontent among those working in the
NHS. This fuels further the feelings of uncertainty. Clinicians
especially voice their concerns at the impact of continuous change
and the managers managing the changes change too often and too
quickly themselves to command credibility. In such a context even
genuine reports of reductions in waiting lists are tainted with

*From Thomas Hobbes (1651) *Leviathan* (1968 edition). Penguin Books,
Harmondsworth, p 185. This classic text of political theory set out the case
for public institutions in society as the basic antidote required to contain
the excesses of human nature.

suspicion, and Ministerial statements about improving Patient's Charter standards are alleged to ring hollow.

The purpose of this book is to help bring clarity where there has been confusion. In 1990 Professor Chris Ham at the University of Birmingham's Health Services Management Centre (HSMC) wrote an excellent account of the NHS reforms designed at the time for an essentially student readership.[1] As it turned out, however, such was the lack of internal clarity in the NHS, even then many managers, clinicians and their professional colleagues kept it on their desks as a vital source of reference and understanding. This book is a similarly short publication and in that it seeks to explain the NHS, a natural successor to *The New National Health Service: organization and management*. Its difference lies, however, in its approach.

FROM PLANNING TO POLITICAL PROCESSES OF DEVELOPMENT

In 1990 it still seemed appropriate to describe the NHS in terms of its structures and strategies. By 1994 'functions' had replaced 'structures' and the Department of Health's organizational chart of the functions in the reformed NHS, reproduced by Professor Ham in his follow-up book very soon became a standard induction and training aid (see Figure 1).[2]

By 1994, however, Ham had replaced 'organization' with 'competition' in his book title and now, three years later, we all have our very different diagrams of today's NHS. As Peter Key and his colleagues' account of *The Unsupported Middle* illustrates so vividly, all maps of the contemporary health care system have become essentially experiential.[3] (Figure 2 provides one graphic example from a Community Health Council perspective.) The task now is to make sense of these; to re-draw the lines of what has become a world which, in Key's memorable phrase, presently has 'oceans without continents'.

This book seeks to explain today's NHS as a political environ-

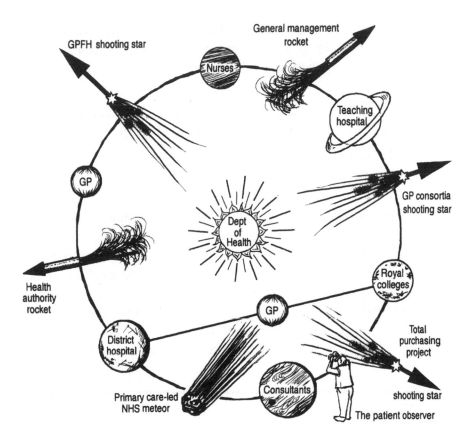

Figure 2: Into the unknown – the 1997 NHS galaxy. As drawn by user and carer representatives at a regional learning event in November 1995.[3]

ment. Its central premise, moreover, is that, with the demise of strategic planning and organizational coherence, the contemporary NHS in terms of its continuing national identity can only be recognized, and its behaviour truly understood, as a political development. The aim is to be authentic; objectivity for the purpose of this particular publication comes second.

The book therefore concentrates on understanding the new relationships of power rather than on the roles of apparent authority. Drawing on a range of experience, both personal and general, it sets out how decision making in the UK health care system now takes place. Its aim is to recognize the realities, to reveal the risks and above all to clarify the opportunities for influence now available to a much wider spectrum of participants in the NHS power-play than was hitherto ever the case.

TRANSLATION OF CONTEMPORARY NHS INTO WIDER UK HEALTH CARE ENVIRONMENT

The exercising of this influence – becoming real contributors to the shaping of health care – is the life blood of the NHS annual cycle. As a matter of basic principle individuals, groups, whole communities always need to be more involved, alongside the established professional bodies and representatives factions. It is upon this involvement and expanded participation that the claims to survival and legitimate primacy of a National Health Service in the UK health care system may well, in the future, substantially depend.

NOTES

1   Ham C (1991) *The New National Health Service: organization and management.* Radcliffe Medical Press, Oxford.

2   Ham C (1994) *Management and Competition in the New NHS.* Radcliffe Medical Press, Oxford. (Second edition is now available)

3   Meads G, Huntington J, Key P *et al.* (1997) *The Unsupported Middle: future developments in a primary care-led NHS.* Radcliffe Medical Press, Oxford.

2

The Balance of Power*

DEVOLUTION AND DIFFERENCE – IMPACT OF GENERAL PRACTICE FUNDHOLDING

As I write these words entries for the seventh wave of general practice fundholding (GPFH) are about to close. It is the 31st day of July 1996 and the last date for those looking to assume control of the purchasing of health care for their practice populations in April 1997, when nationally the level of population coverage is expected to reach 60 per cent. The principle of primary care-led commissioning appears to be irrevocably established in practice, regardless of future changes in national administration, and its expression signifies not simply a new era of *devolution* for the NHS but the sanctioning of *difference* throughout the UK health care system.

As this book proceeds I would like to describe, through these

---

*The Balance of Power was a term coined by the then Prime Minister, Sir Robert Walpole, during a speech to the House of Commons in 1741 and subsequently applied by both political commentators and historians to the equilibrium needed not only within the framework of parliamentary sovereignty in the UK but between the States of Europe in the eighteenth century, and more latterly the international super-powers in present times.

developments, the shift from planning to political processes within the NHS during the 1990s, and the aetiological relationship between these processes and their emerging organizational and service outcomes. In particular, I want to explore the dynamic now created by the abolition of Regional Health Authorities (RHAs) as national policy frameworks and local pressures, personalities and initiatives enter into a new period of direct encounter with one another. The pages that follow describe the passing of the familiar NHS as a much loved national public service institution and yet still anticipate, in the closing chapter of the book, a decade ahead in which NHS strategic priorities can, in my view, be extended more effectively throughout the public and independent sectors than ever before.

This is an important prospect and positive challenge, particularly for those still in direct NHS employment, most of whom are still a long way from being on terms with the continuous changes of the past few years and their significance. Their individual insecurities and collective uncertainty has not equipped them to be ambassadors for the contemporary NHS. The wider public has been left confused; often pleasantly surprised by improved quality and even speed of response, yet at the same time suspicious about motives and in particular that something they owned as precious is now being insidiously privatised.

Which brings us back to general practice fundholding as the exemplary source of this ambivalence. On the one hand, in the face of mounting workload pressures, the popular appreciation of individual general practitioners (GPs) continues to be virtually unrivalled; on the other, the scale and pace of resource transfer to their private businesses is almost unprecedented. In 1997/98 fundholders' income and expenditure for the services they provide and purchase will be over £4 billion, i.e. HCHS/GMS expenditure.

Ten years ago, maybe even five, such a prospect was totally inconceivable. The nature of such change *per se* means that it cannot have been planned, let alone predicted. Development derived from political processes can generate pace but unexpected consequences are part of the deal too. Many of what are now in national terms mainstream service arrangements have been rapidly translated into practice through the successful exercise of informal power. Out-of-hours co-operatives, consortia, and health commissions themselves, are each examples of local developments initially frowned upon as being at the limits of legal discretion which, in a remarkably short space of time, have won such constituencies of support that significant statutory adjustments have been required. In each case the political imperative for change has come from within the informal organization of the NHS, its networks, learning sets and new pressure groups. By comparison the political mandate of parliamentary representatives has appeared at times almost irrelevant.

In terms of the NHS this is a complete about-turn in less than a decade. Ten years ago the NHS could be identified everywhere by the consistency of its structures and its plans. The district general hospital and the general practice were standard models; both often used off-the-shelf kit designs for their buildings. Regional and district plans were of ten and five year durations. Detailed and lengthy, they were underpinned by professional norms, particularly for staffing levels, that applied across the country. Now in 1996/97, as even NHS core values are subtly revised to incorporate *choice* and the consequences of consumerism, what is up for grabs is the extent to which there is any common ground at all nationally. The NHS has become a local creature; the risk, of course, is that in some areas the political processes behind its development could create a local monster (see Figure 3). Politics in any form is a messy business.

Ten years ago I was, almost, still a social worker and the NHS was, almost, still the NHS. Obviously these are simplistically sentimental assertions but it is not just personal nostalgia that fondly recalls a time when the terms 'trust' and 'competition' would rarely have belonged in the same sentence. In 1986 I had only recently begun a career that continues today in the no-man's land between Health and Social Services, having moved from frontline fieldwork where the likes of MIND and MENCAP were still firmly in the role of lobbyists for, and against, those very services for which they are now the chief providers. As a member of local social work teams in Hampshire and Northamptonshire in the 1980s, my number of

NHS Development		
1	Regional and national planning	⟶ local participation, pressure and politics
2	Consensus commitments	⟶ winning constituencies and product champions
3	Intra-NHS	⟶ UK health care system including public and private stakeholders
4	Representative and elected members	⟶ appointees, subsidies and sponsorship
5	Formal	⟶ informal
6	Co-ordinated policy, organizational, managerial, clinical and personal development	⟶ commissioned projects and market fragmentation
7	Specific national strategies	⟶ conceptual central frameworks, e.g. a primary care-led NHS
8	Proactive legislation and parliamentary policy	⟶ reactive statutory adjustments and market regulations
9	Professional and managerial leadership	⟶ commentators, critics and participant observers
10	Standard models	⟶ diversity

Figure 3: The direction of travel, 1990–2000.

admissions to independent residential and nursing homes could easily be counted on the fingers of one hand. By contrast, my counterparts today in many parts of the country are familiar only with such arrangements for their frail elderly and handicapped clients. Ten years ago we all still had door-to-door milkmen and probably most of us thought it would be ever thus. Who would wager today on the survival of the traditional general practice; the very vehicle identified in 1991 for shifting the balance of power in the NHS and now apparently destined, as an organization, to be another casualty of the political change process that it, more than any other agency, helped to trigger?[1]

There is, of course, no shortage of formal explanations for the changes described above. In the peculiar climate of the 1990s when many managers and clinicians alike have sometimes desperately sought for reassurances that they are still doing 'the right thing', these explanations have often come dubiously close to supplying justifications rather than just plain intelligence and understanding. It is not just in the area of clinical research that the academic pursuit of truth has been arguably contaminated by a too close association with contemporary NHS development. There can be a price to pay and that price sometimes is telling it as it is.

SCALE OF NHS INTERNAL CHANGE

The impression of virtual collusion is, of course, at its strongest in official Department of Health versions of events – as indeed, it can be argued, should quite properly be the case – and among the free market theorists whose intellectual contributions were critical to the inception of the reforms. The successors to Marshall Marinker and Alan Enthoven as the gurus of systemic change in the 1990s have learnt that they must be on the inside track of central NHS policy development to be effective.[2] Perhaps not surprisingly therefore the NHSE guidance that the work of such commentators as Carol Propper and Julian Le Grand has spawned remains some of the most theoretically neat but least used documentation in practice at local levels.[3,4] The language of market exits and entries has often felt at best a dangerous diversion to those actually engaged with locally elected representatives and their communities in issues arising from proposed hospital closures or even relatively modest changes of use. At both ends of this spectrum the list of examples continues to grow, from St Bartholomews in London to Odiham Community Hospital in Hampshire, from reducing accident and emergency departments in Newcastle and Bristol to running down a charitable hospital foundation in Suffolk.[5]

The perceived failure of classic organizational theories for public service organizations to make available frameworks that can be applied to the NHS reforms of the 1990s has compounded the collusion. The impact of central communications, the enthusiastic press gained by the minority of today's new health care entrepreneurs, seems almost to have put to flight a generation of NHS apologists which held to the view that normative integration, bureaucratic management models and elected public accountability were together the tripod of organizational principles upon which public services would always depend.[6] Moreover, where classic organizational theories are already on the shelf, available to take off and apply effectively to the contemporary development of an NHS which has increasingly ceased to be a closed system, these are usually derived from studies in the commercial and industrial sectors that, for obvious reasons, the NHS apologists have been extremely reluctant to use. After all, their beliefs in the need for consensus and the professionalization of care were to a large extent counterpoint products to those who defined organizations as fluid coalitions of groups and sub-groups and dynamic fields of forces.[7,8] The conventional wisdom was that those differences were quite simply the distinction between the public and private sectors.

With theory either temporarily on the defensive or permanently discredited, depending upon where you stand, the unhappy impact has been to turn NHS academics from students to commentators. This tendency seems to have been compounded by the number of retired and redundant NHS executives joining the ranks of Visiting Fellows and part-time Professors. Hard research based on actual organizational behaviour has been conspicuous by its absence. The fear factor that has been fundamental in driving through organizational change has unhappily tinged academia as well.

The outcome of this in 1996/97 is the feeling of a depressed NHS with an internal identity crisis and a UK health care system which has felt at times almost anarchic. The relationships of power have threatened to usurp, at least temporarily, roles of authority – but despite the policy rhetoric of a primary care-led NHS it is quite unclear where this power will ultimately rest. In Julian Tudor-Hart's still wonderfully apt phrase, 'not for the last time, doctors claimed territory they were unwilling or unable to occupy' and, as for patients themselves, as close to whom as possible decisions are now meant to be made, the case for their satisfaction remains a tough one to make.[9] Doubling the geographic size of health authorities and the ratcheting up of the performance management levers of central planning priorities point to a rather different direction; few post-1996 health authorities herald themselves as 'people's champions'. The talk now is of 'ringholding' and 'regulation'; terms which themselves testify to the changing nature of both the NHS and the wider UK health care system. Effective contributions to these rely as much on competitive as on vocational motivation. The former requires fair play and constraint; the latter was traditionally the building block of a public service.

ACHIEVING A NEW BALANCE OF POWER

Historically major institutions along with the societies and states they represent must achieve a condition of homeostasis. The mode of control, as in eighteenth century Europe when the phrase 'balance of power' was coined may move from dictatorship to parliamentary sovereignty and back, but for the system to survive shifting power must lead to a new balance. This equilibrium is evidently elusive for an NHS which, as this chapter has explored, is now best understood in behavioural terms as a political process that has deliberately destabilized the established order. Such behaviour is the stuff of revolutions and all revolutions have an end point which, viewed historically, is often abrupt and sudden. Traces of what went before are often hard to detect. The message for many of those seeking to retain a *National* Health Service may be loud and clear; it is counter revolution or bust.

NOTES

1   For a range of alternative organizational and service models in UK primary care, see Meads G (ed.) (1996) *Future Options for General Practice.* Radcliffe Medical Press, Oxford; and Gordon P and Hadley J (eds) (1996) *Extending Primary Care: polyclinics, resource centres, hospitals-at-home.* Radcliffe Medical Press, Oxford.

2   Examples of the mould breaking books and essays that paved the way for the 1990s NHS revolution would include Enthoven A (1985) *Reflections on the Management of the NHS.* Nuffield Provincial Hospitals Trust, London; Marinker M (1984) *Developments in Primary Care* in Teeling Smith G (ed.) *A New NHS Act for 1996?* Office of Health Economics, London; and Marinker M, Maynard A and Pereira Gray D (1986) The doctor, the patient and their contract. *BMJ* **292**: 1438–40.

3 Health economists have played a critical role as both internal contributors and external commentators on the changes in the contemporary
   health care system. Carol Propper from the School of Advanced Urban
   Health Studies at Bristol University, for example, chaired the national
   working party whose report led to HSG (94)55 on the *Operation of
   the NHS Internal Market* (see note 4 below); and Julian Le Grand has
   been a member of the Avon Family Health Services Authority and
   Health Commission who from 1994–96 also played an important role
   regionally in successfully strengthening local GPFH recruitment. A
   typical example of their work together at this time was Propper C, Le
   Grand J and Robinson R (1992) *The Economics of Social Problems.*
   Macmillan, London, and their chapters in Bartlett W and Le Grand J
   (eds) (1993) *Quasi-markets and Social Policy.* Macmillan, London.

4 See NHS Executive (1994) *The Operation of the NHS Internal Market:
   local freedoms, national responsibilities* (HSG (94)55). Department of
   Health, London.

5 See, for example, Hubble D (1997) The East Anglian angle. *Primary
   Care Management* **7**(1): 16.

6 For a classic exposition of the conventional wisdom in terms of
   organizational theory and its application to the public service sector,
   there remains no better book than Etzioni A (1971) *A Comparative
   Analysis of Complex Organizations.* Free Press, New York.

7 See Cyert R and March J (1963) *A Behavioural Theory of the Firm.*
   Prentice-Hall, Englewood Cliffs, New Jersey.

8 See Lewin K (1951) *Field Theory in Social Sciences.* Harper and Row,
   New York.

9 Tudor-Hart J (1988) *A New Kind of Doctor.* Merlin Press, London,
   p 42.

3

Revolution

'Oh! What a revolution!
The age of chivalry is gone. That of sophisters, economists
and calculators, has succeeded.'*

IMPACT OF CHOICE

Although revolutions are not planned they do have an inevitability
about them. They occur when no other means are available to
resolve extreme civil divisions and their outcomes often include the
definition or recreation of nation states. Witness, for example, what
has happened to Yugoslavia in the present decade or go back to
the Russia of 1917, or even the England of 1688. Besides
confirming country boundaries and identities, these latter two also
represented ideological victories, for communism and parliamentary
sovereignty in turn. When great concepts combine with the political
processes unleashed in revolutionary times the force is irresistible.
The democratic ideal was as decisive an outcome as the republican
state for both France and the United States of America – and
thence for much of the western world – of their revolutionary
conditions in the late eighteenth century.

---

*Edmund Burke (1790), the Irish statesman and Whig philosopher, in his
contemporary *Reflections on the Revolution in France*. His political
thought, along with Disraeli's, is regarded as the original source of
modern Conservatism.

The contemporary NHS has felt from the inside as if it is under-going just such a revolutionary period. For 'democracy' substitute 'devolution' and if liberty, fraternity and equality were the ideas that manned the barricades in the 1790s, choice, competition and consumerism could lay claim to being the components of the rallying call to executive arms two hundred years later. Revolutions do not respect geographical boundaries. The ripples of NHS change now reach far and wide. New Zealand has adopted its own versions of general practice fundholding. Even several of the former Soviet satellite states are seeking to introduce their own versions of an internal market in health care, e.g. Poland, Lithuania and Moldova. Commentators offer rational explanations of parallel responses to comparable pressures; but somebody has to start and unequivocally this was the UK in 1990 when the accelerated arrival of purchasing and providing was, significantly, accompanied by the political expressions which are the prerequisites of revolutionary change.[1] There was 'no choice', the public were told; the NHS could not go on any longer as it was. Breaking point had been reached. Even the Presidents of the consultants' Royal Colleges agreed, inadvertently removing the basis for their traditional power by so doing.

But while government proclamations and reforms may start a revolutionary change process, this process itself precludes subse-quent control by any one party. Devolution, like democracy, is not susceptible to top-down delivery. It has to create itself, again and again. The contemporary NHS is in the process of doing just this, and the further this process goes the less the original national blueprint seems to hold sway.

The new theology of the separation of purchasing and providing functions is now blasphemed against by the expanding range of primary managed care organizations that decline to differentiate between the two as they apply the holistic ethos of general practice to commissioning (see Figure 4).[2] These organizations themselves are assuming a range of organizational status that makes the 1990 GMS contract's attempts to confirm the monopoly of the legal partnership in general practice seem now a Canute-like anachronism. NHS trusts geared far more to their own survival than

Type	Purpose	Management	Population
(a) The preferred provider	Transfer of secondary care to community settings under GP control	Locality GP group through which one HA accredited practice purchases on behalf of neighbouring practices and employs or contracts for range of clinicians and HCHS	40 000–80 000; large towns without full DGHs and with range of local premises available
(b) The primary care trust	Community based provider control of local NHS resources and strategy augmented by private finance	Merged general practices and community trust as basis for independent organization along 'Golf Club' lines, with range of membership options and board of stakeholder representatives	100 000 plus; urban areas where GMS underdeveloped and limited premises available
(c) The community care centre	Provides a major unified resource for information, support and advice to exploit local potential for self-help	Centre management group includes user representatives with a strong patients' association, integrated GPFH and SSD budgets and proprietary links to local residential and day care units	15 000–35 000 small towns, suburbs with large established general practices

Figure 4: Primary managed care: organizational options.[2]

that of the NHS, under cost and clinical pressures, increasingly expand their income streams to the point where the NHS prefix seems almost a misnomer. Add in the mixed economy now represented by general dental and optometric services and the organizational variety brought about by the 1990s health care revolution is clear. Local people are doing their own thing. If the time arrives when, as a national institution, it is held together by the names on its payroll – and many of these are now there as sub-contractors – its own status will be in trouble.

IMPLICATIONS FOR PUBLIC ACCOUNTABILITY OF NHS STRUCTURAL CHANGE

In structural terms the management basis for devolution in the NHS has been the adoption of a standard population based funding formula for nationwide application. This has permitted the progressive transfer of responsibility for funding decisions and with each transfer the framework for public accountability has radically altered. The pre-1990 NHS now seems deceptively simple and straightforward. Parliamentary accountability and the central mechanism for differential allocations, called the RAWP (Resource Allocation Working Party) formula, went together. Ministers were directly answerable for decisions taken throughout the NHS and this NHS essentially meant hospitals and their associated catchment area services.

From 1990 to 1995 during the sea change to community care RHAs applied the new weighted capitation formula with sometimes as much as a 10 per cent differential between health authorities as they took into effect the variable impact of such factors as 'free good' military hospitals, long stay institutional closures and teaching units. Their members were the appointed agents of this strategic change, swiftly set aside once primary care-led purchasing had taken root.

On 31 March 1994, with six months notice, 14 RHAs were brought to a summary conclusion. For some, such as Wessex and Yorkshire where the concept and practice of 'health commissions' had been pioneered, there was the sudden dawning for many staff that they had been agents of their own destruction. And the suicide ratio was high; regional payrolls were reduced from up to 1000 to just over 100 in the creation of eight new RHAs, with a strictly time limited life expectancy.

On 31 March 1996 these too were terminated. Separate public accountability at the level between a national headquarters for a population of 60 million and the local district was gone; and this regional level covering as it did, on average, around 7 million inhabitants, was equivalent to half the countries in modern Europe. The pace and scale of change was revolutionary, but so too more significantly was the effect on 'development' itself.

SUBSIDIARITY AND DEVELOPMENT

Subsidiarity is a splendid principle and an expedient one. Few in the UK will not be familiar with its use by national politicians in the mid-1990s to justify the retention of national controls in the face of often pan-EU opposition. It has been a convenient communications aid and, above all, a means of retaining broad based conservative support, including sometimes even those with more xenophobic tendencies. But subsidiarity and strategy are uneasy bedfellows. They may read well together but, in practice, that is about as far as it goes. Development derived from strategy, however flawed or fallible, is a very different product or indeed, range of products, to those spawned by converting the principle of subsidiarity into practice.

This change is central to the contemporary NHS revolution. Development has many dimensions – managerial, clinical, professional, organizational and personal – to name but five, and these are no longer co-ordinated. Each now progresses at its own different pace, locally, or not at all. With the demise of RHAs there is not only no locus for their integration but no agency responsible even for commissioning their co-ordination. The new regional offices of the NHS Executive do not have funds for the task. It is not part of their terms of reference; performance management has often become synonymous with monitoring. NHS development belongs in the universities, with the consultancies, and at the doorstep of general practices and providers themselves.

The problem with this is that many of these are either only dimly aware of these changes or, even where they are more or less up to speed on the policy agenda, ill equipped to respond. *Development itself needs developing.* It is not an automatic function and the incentives for responding to the present revolutionary changes are not great. Why change educational curricula today when tomorrow the policy priorities may well dramatically shift again? Many hospitals, medical schools and universities are more than just closely aligned. Their very survival depends upon one another and universities over the centuries, in particular, have a history of sitting tight and successfully seeing through revolutionary times.

The NHS of 1997 is not like Paris of 20 years ago. Its students will not be on the streets for a primary care-led NHS. I found when I addressed the NHS National Trainees conference in February 1996 that, in a show of hands, only three out of the approximately two hundred people present in the audience intended to start their careers with general practices. The use of a simple self-assessment tool at local NHS seminars, in terms of readiness for its primary care-led policy, has produced some predictably low scores (see Figure 5), not least among the managers and staff of NHS community trusts who might have been expected to do better. The

---

Please give yourself an honest score of between 1 and 10 on each of the following, with higher scores indicating strengths.

Score

(i)   A background in community based services
(ii)   Involvement with primary care teams
(iii) Understanding of Family Health Services Contracts
(iv)   Contribution to health and social services collaboration
(v)   Work with independent sector
(vi)   Support for development of primary care-led purchasing
(vii) Service shifts from secondary care
(viii) Participation in inter-professional education
(ix)   Practising devolved responsibility to patients
(x)   Commitment to primary care-led NHS policy

(Any scores over 70 require validation by a viva!)

Figure 5:   Preparing for a primary care-centred NHS: self-assessment test.

identification of the NHS with secondary care institutions, however, conditions us all.

This institutional conditioning of the NHS and its historic allies still runs deep. The revolution may be heading in a direction where hospitals turn into local facilities on, for example, a city-wide health campus – where the medical principles of general practice convert into the wider ethic of personal care management – but we are as yet a long way from systematically developing the people and programmes to serve in this post-revolutionary era. For the present decade at least the revolutionary process goes on.

NOTES

1   Helpful accounts of parallel international developments in health care systems are contained, for example, in Fry J and Horder J (1994) *Primary Health Care in an International Context.* Nuffield Provincial Hospitals Trust, London; Ham C (1994) *Management and Competition in the New NHS.* Radcliffe Medical Press, Oxford, pp 56–60. On lessons from poorer countries see Macdonald J (1992) *Primary Health Care: preventing medicine.* Earthsea Publications, London.

2   Meads G (1996) Future options for general practice. *British Journal of Health Care Management* **2**(7): 372–4.

4

The Dark Ages

'They plundered all the neighbouring cities and country, spread the conflagration from the eastern to the western sea, without any opposition, and covered almost every part of the devoted island. Public as well as private structures were overturned.'*

DECLINE IN NHS STANDARDS OF BEHAVIOUR AND MORALE

There are times best forgotten and perhaps, fortuitously, these are often the times about which least is known. Progress and information go well together. Destructive behaviour and sound record keeping are inimical. For the NHS of the 1990s this has been literally true. The passing of over 400 statutory organizations in the space of five years has witnessed warehouses of archives pile up and pass silently away. Research has almost by default, become exclusively clinical. The rapidity of organizational and personnel change has meant that time after time even medium term evaluation studies have been shot away by the summary removal of the assumptions on which they were based. And to whom would their

---

*The great monastic scholar, The Venerable Bede, describes the impact of the invasion by the Anglo Saxons and Jutes between AD 450–456 at the start of the Dark Ages in Britain, in *The Ecclesiastical History of the English Nation*. Everyman Edition (1965), London, p 23.

outcomes be reported? It seems as if a whole generation has been lost to the NHS. Fifty is now the unofficial standard retirement age for senior management. Only the exceptions seem to survive longer. For many these are the dark ages; the NHS which is increasingly called upon to meet the demographic care challenge of increases in its frail elderly population responds by removing all but the relatively young, fit and mobile from within its own ranks.

The Dark Ages of history are those where the sense of society no longer holds sway. Civilization ceases to exist; competing interests strive not simply for control but to eradicate each other, and different tribes and cultures vie for ultimate supremacy. These are the times of pillaging and philandering, when the overarching values of law and order no longer function without the need for formidable force.

A NEW PARADIGM OF PUBLIC ACCOUNTABILITY

The demise of traditional public accountability structures in the NHS of the 1990s represents for many its 'dark ages'. The aggressive tribalism of its medical, financial, nursing and (increasing number of) para-medical professions has never been so much in evidence. Having been confined in the past to the inner sanctum of Department of Health meeting rooms, conflicts of interest have never been so visible locally. The feuds are played out across the overlapping health care markets which now make up the NHS. Furthermore, not only are there more disputes actually built into the pattern of NHS transactions – see Figure 6 which analyses the HA/GPFH axis at the root of these – there are also many more tribes eager to exploit, for example, the advent of local pay bargaining and the decline of the central collegiate negotiating machinery. Different types of physiotherapists, for example, out in the community have increased by two-thirds over five years; alternative therapists abound and, in the face of all logic, nursing continues to divide itself into ever more specialisms.

Health authorities	versus	GPFHs
Population based and community oriented	v.	Oriented to individuals, families and special needs
Focus on overall health needs	v.	Driven by patient demand
Salaried staff usually on permanent contracts	v.	Self-employed reliance on annual business dividend
Secure sources of recurrent NHS capital and revenue	v.	Variable income levels from range of contracts including insurance companies, occupational health schemes and bank overdrafts
Funding via weighted capitation formulae	v.	Motivated financially by achieving higher volumes of fees, allowances and screening targets, with GPFH allocations based on historic patterns of HCHS usage
Employee status staff and management with frequently changing functions lack real sense of ownership of health authorities	v.	Power and money belongs to the practices where professional roles and responsibilities are relatively constant
Long history of working with local authorities, often unproductively and sometimes collusively	v.	Often an anathema historically to local authorities whose councellors are now threatened by loss of control inherent in GPFH/care management alliances and devolved budgets
Belong to modern EU political culture of (sub) regional strategic planners	v.	Characteristic of UK political culture of the new consumerism
Appointed statutory membership represents traditional public authority and accountability	v.	Popular support and patient 'stakeholders' offer democratic alternative to legitimize public services
Can be perceived as remote from the public they claim to champion	v.	In daily contact with users and carers, 24-hour access
Have required regular and detailed performance management rather than regulation	v.	Entrepreneurial businesses, privately owned, fit for the (health care) market place
Report to intermediate tier via formal chains of command and management channels	v.	Direct access to Department of Health and ministerial response of GPFH/GMSC leadership
Identified with long waiting lists, hospital crises and low efficiency	v.	Unprecedented levels of planned savings, prescribing underspends and 100 per cent targets achievements
Purchasing has, so far, served risk management and cost containment rather than real health gain or general shifts from acute care	v.	Really promote primary care and serve as a vehicle for central policy in aligning providers with health objectives
Regarded by many as a transitional organizational phase en route to universal primary care-led purchasing	v.	Here to stay: yesterday, today and tomorrow

Figure 6: The commissioning contest. (Source: Meads G (1994) *Primary Care Management* **4**(3): 2.)

The national rallying cry of a 'primary care-led NHS' should be a unifying force, but there are now few leaders in position to take up the call.[1] Sadly it seems the new regional Chairs will virtually be discounted by the external NHS; their role, with the best will in the world, appears an impossible one. Widely seen as the symbols of central patronage they relate to 600 plus members and 60 odd Chairs, each now looking locally for their essential legitimacy.

And to many the Chairs of the remaining rump of post-1996 health authorities appear in the darkest conditions of all. Saddled with support, strategy and monitoring as their basic but often seemingly incompatible core responsibilities, they are now expected to be the frontline local agents of the national leadership.[2] But more often than not they are no such thing. They lack not just the money and mechanisms but, more importantly, the history for the task. General management and general practice do not have a history of getting along well with each other. The latter has always known it has the option of sitting tight. Until now at least it could always be sure of outlasting the seemingly ever changing health authority. Indeed rooting the reforms of 1990 in general practice with its apparently certain continuity, was originally one of the great attractions for central government. But now both are in the political frontline. Local primary care contracts and alternative providers (see Figure 4, p 17) are in the offing and survival is suddenly a common cause. The scale of the targets for 'overhead' reductions that all national political parties espouse offers no immunities.[3] 'Downsizing' and 'rationalization' are euphemisms that apply to all parts of the UK health care system; NHS trusts emerge; BUPA cuts its hospitals and sponsors its own general practices; single handed GPs appear increasingly an anachronism and even hospices struggle for their revenue funding.

Who needs who most in these conditions? Why should general practice look to a local health authority for development as well as monitoring; to give with the one hand while taking rather more with the other? Competitive purchasing, with health authorities pitted not simply against fundholders, in their various guises, but against one another remains the most obvious route available to tackle excessive transaction costs. And general practice has plenty

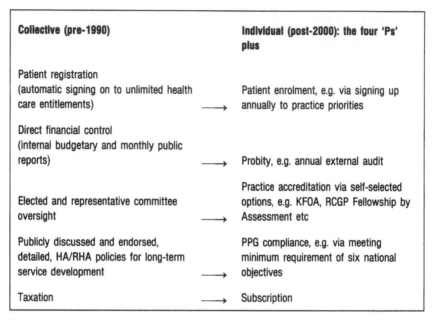

Collective (pre-1990)	Individual (post-2000): the four 'Ps' plus
Patient registration (automatic signing on to unlimited health care entitlements) ⟶	Patient enrolment, e.g. via signing up annually to practice priorities
Direct financial control (internal budgetary and monthly public reports) ⟶	Probity, e.g. annual external audit
Elected and representative committee oversight ⟶	Practice accreditation via self-selected options, e.g. KFOA, RCGP Fellowship by Assessment etc
Publicly discussed and endorsed, detailed, HA/RHA policies for long-term service development ⟶	PPG compliance, e.g. via meeting minimum requirement of six national objectives
Taxation ⟶	Subscription

Figure 7:   The changing paradigm of public accountability.

of other options open to it in terms of potential development agencies willing to support its position in the vanguard of change. Pharmaceutical facilities companies already sponsor disease management and managed care projects and pay for a large part of the postgraduate education programme; banks underwrite practice premises and such corporate enterprises as the International Hospitals Group and major insurance companies like the Norwich Union are already putting out financial feelers, waiting in the wings ready to invest further in an NHS health care market where not just stability but growth of consumer demand is virtually guaranteed.

These are not the conditions in which a new paradigm of public accountability can simply be left to emerge. It is not, of course, difficult to detect what its component parts might be: probity, practice accreditation, patient enrolment and basic compliance with national planning priorities (the four 'Ps'; see Figure 7). But this framework is in its infancy. In its place still is direct parliamentary accountability for the NHS as a whole without adequate designated responsibilities for its parts. The Hansards of 1995/96 are littered with unanswered questions and stock (non) replies: 'This information/decision is no longer collected/taken centrally'. But nor are they anywhere else. Predictably, health authorities try to turn the clocks back with, for instance, commissioning 'localities', from Devon to Dundee, resembling the old areas in all but name.

And it is the name and what it signifies that is important. Co-ordinated commissioning offers a degree of managerial control but the term 'Area Health Authority', for example, provides a structure of elected and representative committees that the products of consumerism have yet to begin to challenge. In the Dark Ages people simply behave less well; they look (even) more to their own interests than to others. There are no custodians of the overall public interest and a health care system which becomes increasingly based upon the principle of individual need can itself start to become little more than the aggregate of its individuals' interests. Which teams have endured in the contemporary NHS, let alone organizations? Whose contract term has been lengthened not shortened? Who is not aware, all the time, of his or her redundancy package? The answers are 'very few' if my NHS experience of the past five years is a reliable guide. Loyalty and reciprocal respect are the chief casualties.

Moreover a sizeable chunk of this experience of mine was actually as an NHS Director of Performance Management in the South and West region. I entered the role talking of the need for integration; of quality with quantity, of development and monitoring, of fusing the top-down and bottom-up. I left having learnt the language of efficiency and effectiveness; too often historically the trademarks of a totalitarian regime when applied to the exclusion of all else.

I also left with the new 1997 Primary Care Bill in the offing, designed to further cement the devolutionary process for financial control, service development and clinical priority setting in the NHS. Self-determination is one important principle right at the heart of the process. It is an attractive principle offering the prospect of moving away from the dependency culture and paternalism that has traditionally plagued the NHS. Its practice depends on us operating maturely in what social psychologists have termed

(a) **Pre-1990s: familial**
    Parent ⟶ Child, e.g. consultants to patients, DHA to CHC
    Child ⟶ Parent, e.g. NHS to Department of Health, FHS contractors to FHSA/FPC

(b) **1990s: immature/transitional**
    Child ⟶ Adult, e.g. HAs in deficit with NHSE regional offices, new PCTs with HAs
    Adult ⟶ Parent, e.g. trusts with HAs, NHSE with DoH

(c) **Post-1990s: mature/prospective**
    Adult ⟷ Adult, e.g. HA/GPFH strategic alliances, preferred provider long-term service agreements, RO market regulation, GP/patient priority setting

Figure 8: The NHS relationships set.

an adult–adult relationship; whether as professional to patient, management to staff or commissioner-to-contractor (see Figure 8).[4]

But the role models do not yet exist. The internal NHS has become conditioned to conflict. Despite the worthy efforts of such authorities in the South and West as Dorset, Somerset and South-ampton, and to a lesser extent elsewhere, with their comprehensive health care management programmes, e.g. for coronary heart disease, running in parallel with the contracting cycle; *collaboration* has often become a stranger.[5] Even *partnership*, the very essence and standard organizational unit of general practice, the traditional bedrock of the NHS, is now under threat. The new primary care legislation seems surely bound to usher in wave upon wave of locally piloted, nationally sanctioned, different types of primary care organizations (see Figure 4, p 17). Regulating these hybrids, often without rules, seems now to be the future destiny of today's diminished health authorities.

THE SPIRITUAL DIMENSION

Partnership and collaboration are the spirit of relationships turned into form. The spiritual void is ultimately the defining dimension of the Dark Ages. Not that NHS based chaplains are not busy. The expansion in their numbers has been one of the apparent surprises of the present decade, although clearly not entirely divorced as a development from the internal NHS casualty rate resulting from the scale and pace of recent organizational change.[6] Health care with its essential healing element is as much a spiritual experience as it is a technical activity. The relationship between people at times of illness or disadvantage is profoundly personal. It depends crucially on their feelings and the values they bring to the encounter. The efficacy of care itself relies on the nature of this relationship; a relationship that is founded in individual, organizational and societal values of generosity and common fellowship.

In the Dark Ages in England a few monasteries kept the flame flickering for such principles as the Nordic invaders spoilt the lands about them. We still read the writings of The Venerable Bede today, a standard text for the university historian and an enduring testimony to the strength of the human spirit in troubled times. Medieval history tells of the Dark Ages coming to a close through a curious combination of popular reaction and external conquest from mainland Europe. It now seems that the future of the NHS may well be determined through the interplay of the modern counterparts of these very same forces.

NOTES

1   The policy direction determined by the term a 'primary care-led NHS' was effectively defined by the NHS Executive in October 1994 through its EL (94)79 *Developing NHS Purchasing and GP Fundholding: towards a primary care-led NHS*. Department of Health, London. This has been followed by a range of managerial and ministerial communications including, of most significance, a members' briefing pack (November 1995), and the Secretary of State for Health, the Rt Hon. Stephen Dorrell's report on the 1995/96 national 'listening exercise' on how to take forward primary care development: NHSE (1996) *Primary Care: the future*. Department of Health, London.

2   Statement to House of Commons by Secretary of State for Health, Rt Hon. Virginia Bottomley on 'Managing the new NHS', 21 October 1993.

3 For 1996/97 the government required an overall 5 per cent reduction in NHS management costs, with no uplift for inflation from 1995/96. At its annual conference in October 1996, the Labour Party then announced that, if elected, it would seek a further £100m reduction to assist in funding its policy of further reducing waiting times, particularly for patients with cancer.

4 See, for example, Bion W (1961) *Experience in Groups.* Tavistock, London; and Berne E (1968) *Games People Play: the psychology of human relationships.* Penguin, Harmondsworth.

5 Oxfordshire is just one excellent and prize winning example of the growing number of effective health care management programmes now being pursued by local health authorities. See O'Brien M and Warren V (1994) What the doctor ordered. *Health Service Journal* **104** (5402): 27, and the reports on the HSJ 1996 Purchaser awards that also included Lanark and Somerset in the *Health Service Journal* (1996) **106** (5530).

6 Dix A (1996) Is God good value? *Health Service Journal* **106** (5511): 24–7.

5

Counter Revolution

'When the Committee saw to it that Robespierre should be outlawed by the Parliament, they knocked away, without knowing it, the keystone of their own policy; it was his popular position which made their policy possible. When he was destroyed they suddenly found that the Terror could no longer be maintained.'*

EUROPEAN INFLUENCES

Those who begin a revolution do not finish it. More often than not they do not even survive to be there at the end. The NHS of the 1990s is peopled with its local Robespierres – the entrepreneurial fundholder, the charismatic chief executive – but has yet to find its Napoleon. Those who seek to raise a popular outcry against the

*From Hilaire Belloc (1966 edn, first published 1911) *The French Revolution*. Oxford University Press, London, p 42. Maximilien Marie Isidore de Robespierre (1758–94) was the Public Accuser in the early phase of the French Revolution, admired for his incorruptibility, as he confronted royalist members of the Assembly appointed by Louis XVI. A Jacobin, he became virtually the ruler of France in 1794 after the King's execution, only to fall foul of the Girondist majority in the Committee of Public Safety which he himself had helped to create. He was sent to the guillotine on 28 July 1794.

Ancien Regime are usually consumed by the violence they believed they could control. Conflict spreads in all kinds of unexpected, unpredictable ways and eventually the public reaction is to revert to a new conservatism, to rally against the spectre of a common enemy and to seek salvation in a new established order.

An internally divided contemporary NHS with its contracting disputes, arbitrations and array of potential conflict mechanisms seems frequently to be searching for its common enemy. Nowadays there can surely only be one candidate! Given its unique relationship with and within both central government and society at large, it has to be Europe. The threat of EU regulations being imposed on the customs of NHS practice may well be enough to trigger a popular call to arms. The reassertion of an NHS collective identity, albeit with different structures and processes to those which applied in the pre-1990 era, can follow given a political leadership capable of capturing public confidence and the changing mood. There is no sign that people will tolerate any threat to the monopoly of general practice through attempts to apply EU service tendering regulations; they seem bound to object to Dutch or even Swedish style subscription systems and they are determined to preserve the international leadership of such NHS home-grown products as professional training, primary care 'gatekeepers' and pharmaceutical licensing programmes.[1] It could be 1066 all over again; the Dark Ages finally ended by a cross-Channel conquest which yet came to signal a national rebirth.

As this implies, external influences already are and will continue to be far reaching in their influence: on procurement procedures, health and safety standards, capital investment, drugs misuse prevention programmes and many other areas. But ultimately the European point of reference is now to help an island's National Health Service define what it is not; a vital offering in times when, as described in the previous chapters, its new political development processes have the potential to pursue difference and diversity to the point where overall policy direction becomes an irrelevance. Polyclinics, private insurance, state hospitals, internists and multi-tier ambulance services are not for us. UK health care at its heart

remains unchanged. On the one hand, for the UK, the NHS epito-
mises its sense of collective responsibility. On the other, the GP
personifies its essential personal values and relationships. The latter
cannot *per se* be tarnished by money. That would be a contradiction in terms. And so the NHS must be paid for by us all, through
national taxation, to permit this established order to remain.

The policy of creating a more primary care-centred health system
in the UK needs to be understood in this context. Both the main
political parties support this policy with commentators noting a
great deal of sophistry in the alleged differences of their 1996 and
1997 pre-election statements.[2] The gaps between local GP commissioning groups, GPFH consortia and multi-funds are hard to detect.
The common underlying principle is that of gaining greater local
ownership of the NHS, with the general practitioner as the standard
proxy for the patient.

CONSUMERIST INFLUENCES

It is here that the counter revolution begins. The starting point is
always when the individual is taken for granted. Revolutionary
leaders who have championed 'the common man' have all too
often discovered to their discomfort that such an individual, if he
exists, does so in his, or just as likely her, own right, with clear
views on the subject of self-interest. The parallel is the so-called
'consumer' of the contemporary NHS. Central NHS Executive
Planning Priorities contain seductively attractive phrases and not a
few weasel, if well-intentioned words, on the subject of a primary
care-led NHS.[3] Indeed, I have written many myself! The promise is
that it will ensure not just the better co-ordination of care but
more sensitive care processes and even decision making as close to
the patient as possible. It sounds good.

But it also sometimes sounds false. As Fedelma Winkler, in a
recent classic essay has beautifully argued, the equity which the
NHS requires is intrinsically at odds with the diversity of general
practice, given a structure of primary care in the UK which permits
9000 small businesses to largely determine themselves the different

levels of services they will provide.[4] Winkler argues persuasively for a franchising model to address what she describes as an inverse relationship between needs and resources in primary care, and advocates powerfully for less proxy and more direct patient involvement. Her hope that strategic planning and co-ordination may be the sources of such changes seems, however, less likely to be fulfilled, given the developmental processes now at play throughout the NHS, than the rather cruder effect of patient responses to the new demand control requirements of a primary care-led NHS.

DEMAND PRESSURES

Like all revolutions the NHS revolution is not living up to all of its original promises. Speed of access has improved, reception areas are smarter, Patient's Charter-conscious staff seem more courteous, but waiting lists are now stuck and in some cases, in 1996/97, actually moving upwards beyond 12 months. Variations between districts continue to be extreme, particularly as both surgical procedures and their outcomes are much more visible through newspapers and performance tables. So too are the costs. A degree of disillusionment is unavoidable. Disaffected people turn to the general practice as they have always done. Weekly magazines, radio phone-ins, the Health Education Authority and health and fitness studios all point in the same direction; and many of the recently built, newly titled GP resource or community centres represent alternative venues for the giving and receiving of all kinds of advice.

But the demand is too much. A primary care-led NHS had as its policy sub-agenda priority setting for secondary care. In November 1996 at their Annual Course in Glasgow, the 150 members of the Association of Managers in General Practice (AMGP) present were more concerned with looking at ten alternative future techniques for constraining demand in primary care (see Figure 9). When I talked with them it was plain to see that having, for the most part, given up on both of the customary central VFM panaceas, in terms of either improved resource allocations or utilization, they were

Within the context of contemporary NHS policy and values the following are suggested as a range of methods local practices might apply to cope with increasing workload pressures, either by containing and redirecting demand or increasing the supply of services. The basic assumption, of course, is finite resources which are perceived as insufficient.

Using a 1–10 scale, with 10 signifying the most preferred option, please score the following ten techniques in terms of their potential use in legitimizing the 'rationing process'.

(i) **Patient enrolment**, e.g. personal registration fee, annual subscriptions etc

(ii) **Patient education**, e.g. on areas for self-care, alternative services etc

(iii) **Reduced access**, e.g. fewer surgery times, rationalized number of service outlets

(iv) **Substitution**, e.g. use of nurse practitioners, counsellors etc

(v) **Triage**, e.g. frontline triage nurses, telephone helplines etc

(vi) **Stakeholding**, e.g. agreed priorities with patient representatives or local authority councellors

(vii) **Joint ventures**, e.g. assuming charitable trust or limited company status, combining with retail pharmacies or insurance companies etc, to extend income and capital base for more services

(viii) **Fees for services**, e.g. charges for 'non-essential' services, self-inflicted conditions etc

(ix) **Insurance**, i.e. shift from public taxation to personal insurance based NHS, still as a universal scheme but with classified hierarchies of conditions

(x) **Private practice**, i.e. opt-out from NHS Terms of Service and reliance on local and individual contracts based on self-determined priorities

Figure 9: Practice techniques for priority setting.

looking to address the rationing issue head on at home, i.e. in their own local surgeries.

To do this they need popular backing and certainly not just via tokenistic patient participation groups. To be successful they need patients to take charge themselves and, in some circumstances, to be prepared to change themselves. The practice managers left Glasgow newly aware of their part in the political development processes of the contemporary NHS. Their future practice leaflets can be thought of as tomorrow's local NHS manifestos representing the pledges of what care will and will not be both provided and commissioned. The patient registration may well be transformed from a signature to a ballot box style sign of support for a local package of practice policies and priorities. Above all the meaning of 'partnership' must change; not just from uni- to inter-professional but to a real practical alliance of patients and practitioners, of formal and informal carers, of those who will pay their way not just for themselves but for the whole practice population.

This is the counter revolution of the late 1990's in the NHS which is underway. As in Paris 200 years ago, the capital and its insurgents have become tired and short on new ideas. It is out in the country that the revolutionary ripples are now to be felt to best effect. Witness, for example, Lyme Regis and Yaxley where the practices already operate as if locally owned, with the most radical and readily accepted service reprofiling as a result.[5,6] Downsizing and development together is a hard trick to pull off. Conjuring with the new forces of this counter revolution requires a renaissance in learning and culture if the old NHS is to emerge renewed.

NOTES

1 See section 4 in Fry J and Horder J (1994) *Primary Health Care in an International Context.* Nuffield Provincial Hospitals Trust, London, pp 64–71, 77–83.

2 The extent to which there is common ground between Conservative and Labour health and health care policies has been particularly well described in Klein R (1996) Labour's draft manifesto: a triumph of style over matter. *BMJ* **13**: 68 and Mankin P (1996) Clearing a path towards a primary care-led NHS. *Primary Care Management* **6**(3): 3–6.

3 Having helped with the initial drafting, I am very understanding of the extent to which the final PPG have to be committee products. The need to balance and include different interests is always captured in the supplementary and sub-clauses. The following 1997/98 example in relation to a primary care-led NHS illustrates this beautifully. From Medium Term Priority A:

> 'A3. Each Health Authority should have agreed with practices their key development needs and the priorities for support required to address them including education and staffing; and should have developed jointly with GPs equitable arrangements for allocating resources and (particularly with GP fundholders) for managing financial risk'. EL (96)45, NHSE, p 12.

4 Winkler F (1996) *Collective and individual responsibilities,* in Meads

G (ed.) *A Primary Care-Centred NHS: the lead phase.* Churchill Living-stone, London, pp 2–8.

5 Dr Barry Robinson, in my view, is the foremost innovator today in terms of the organization of primary care. See Robinson B (1993) Lyme cordial. *Health Service Journal* **103**: 20–2 and Robinson B (1994) Integrating health and social care: the Lyme Community Care Unit. *Community Care Management and Planning* **2**(5): 139–43.

6 Dr Tom Davies, the son of a Liverpool Director of Social Services and former RCGP 'lead' Council member on community care, has helped create a general practice near Peterborough which serves as a multi-faceted resource centre for a wide range of local community needs. See Davies T (1996) *The GP based care network*, in Meads G (ed.) *Future Options for General Practice.* Radcliffe Medical Press, Oxford.

6

Renaissance

'Because truth and social authority were bound together,
knowledge was politics. Any challenge to the traditional world-
view was implicitly a challenge to those who held power in
society, and so inevitably involved a power-struggle.'*

LEADERSHIP BY PARTICIPANT OBSERVERS IN THE NHS

As the NHS translates itself into the wider UK health care system,
creative responses to internally intractable problems increasingly
come from those operating at its interfaces. Health and health care
leadership is more and more provided by those moving to semi-
detached positions, capable of combining a cluster of roles which
legitimize loyalty to the NHS with construction and criticism
together. The renaissance of the NHS, through the renewed local
ownership described in the previous chapter, depends upon its
new breed of participant observers. Mainstream operational
managers are under too much pressure. Academics seem

---

*With these words, Don Cupitt, the contemporary Cambridge theologian
and broadcaster, prefaces his description of Galileo's challenge to the
conventional understanding of the workings of the universe in the late
sixteenth century, during which period his relationship with the Catholic
church was deeply ambivalent. In Cupitt D (1984) *The Sea of Faith*. BBC,
London.

somewhere else; distant, preoccupied with fundamental changes in their own institutions and left behind by the pace and peculiarities of the political development processes that now hold sway in the NHS. They search desperately to fit these into tidy theoretical frameworks for a New Liberalism. Politicians are otherwise engaged and starved of both intelligence and information as the long term central goal of detaching the Executive of the NHS from the Westminster arena incrementally comes to pass. No, the renaissance of the NHS is being left to its local activists.

This, however, does not mean that discrete financial patronage does not have its part to play. Indeed patronage is a more prominent component of the contemporary NHS in which all non-executive board memberships are by appointment and much executive recruitment is by recommendation. The creativity of the art of Michelangelo and Leonardo da Vinci did not simply change the course of history; together they and the schools of learning to which they gave rise re-created the terms on which society existed. So too arguably did the music of Mozart and Beethoven three centuries later. In each case aristocratic or royal patronage was a prerequisite. The NHS today is being fundamentally changed by those local leaders who have and can retain the tacit support of the establishment. They tread a tightrope, sustaining and significantly shifting the status quo at one and the same time, never being quite certain for how long their star will be in the ascendancy, for NHS patronage today can often be rather fickle and transitory.

MODERN UK HEALTH CARE LEADERS AND THEIR METHODS

Take Ian Carruthers and Brian Edwards. At district and regional levels respectively they can fairly be said to have contributed as much as any two individuals to the future renaissance of the NHS. Without them and their groundwork it is hard to conceive of the conditions in which a primary care-led national policy initiative could have been conceived. Like all those blessed historically with the genius of renaissance, in their own times the critics have been as abundant as the copyists. But all have been influenced, and everywhere it will never be the same again.

The local NHS can be reborn because of the creative triumphs of Dorset and the Midlands, where Ian and Brian have been Chief Executives throughout the 1990s, and much more besides. Both are the individuals who have been, *par excellence*, the master managerial politicians of their age, completely attuned to the vicissitudes of the times. And both have been participant observers. Ian Carruthers combines his role as a health authority general manager with two part-time Visiting Fellowships, at the King's Fund College in London and Manchester University. The latter constitute around 25 per cent of his formal working commitments. These are far more than a future retirement option or a safe haven for progressive thinking, they are actually a genuine locus for leadership in today's increasingly pluralistic health care environment.

Brian Edwards moved completely into academia at Sheffield University in April 1996, building on the Visiting Professorship role he had previously occupied alongside his successive posts of Regional General Manager of the Trent and West Midlands Regional Health Authorities during the 1990s. Such a combination clearly helped strengthen his hand as these regions became the pioneers of performance tables and the Patient's Charter. The same was true for Carruthers as he created the first effective health commission, health plans and models of primary care-led purchasing in the UK; and he was astute enough to locate the pilot sites as far away from the central gaze as possible, across the ferry to Swanage, beyond the cliffs at Lyme Regis, in the depths of the New Forest at Verwood.[1]

This exploitation of the new development potential at the local boundaries of the NHS – epitomized by Edwards' regular public platform anecdotes about the fictitious downtrodden working class 'Mrs Smith' – saw Messrs Edwards, Carruthers and their disciples work the informal organization of the 1990s NHS for all it was worth. And in terms of making things happen, it has been worth a great deal. Membership, in Carruthers case, of the central DoH/ NHSE working groups for Health of the Nation, Purchaser Development and the Functions and Manpower Review (FMR) between 1990 and 1994, with even a spell as locum Regional Director thrown in during 1994/95, has counted for far less than the countless societies, associations, networks, clubs, dinners and learning sets addressed during this period. In terms of challenging the conventions of the NHS as a national institution it has been tantamount to guerrilla warfare.

This renaissance has had its parallels among the professional leadership of the 1990s where, for political touch, even Carruthers and Edwards have been put in the shade by the likes of Sir Donald Irvine. Modestly claiming all the time that he is just a humble GP from Ashington in Northumberland, Sir Donald has seemingly effortlessly combined this vocation, since the late 1980s, with Presidency of the Royal College of General Practitioners (RCGP), an association with the King's Fund and, finally, no less than the Chairmanship of the General Medical Council (GMC) itself. With each move, a major legacy: a new GP contract rooted in health promotion; the production of medical audit swiftly turning into cross-sectoral clinical audit; and finally, for the first time, practice accreditation. And, of course, Sir Donald is a first wave fundholder as well; truly the professional renaissance man in contemporary terms.

There are plenty of others too; for example, Patrick Pietroni, London GP in downtown Marylebone occupying the crypt of a church and Postgraduate Dean and occupant of a Chair at Westminster University. Professor Pietroni, together with Donald Irvine, has helped to subtly redefine the role of primary care in relation to secondary care on behalf of the whole practice popula-

---

- To provide care of good quality to individual patients
- To improve the health of the practice population
- To secure secondary care of good quality for individual patients, when required
- To promote learning, teaching and research

Figure 10: Sir Donald Irvine's different kind of future practice, future core functions. (Source: Irvine D and Irvine S (1996) *The Practice of Quality.* Radcliffe Medical Press, Oxford, p 25.)

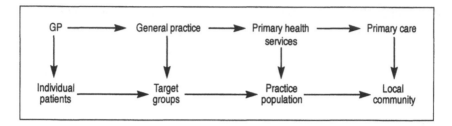

Figure 11: The changing focus – 1990 to 2000.

tion, emphasizing a self-educative model for the future quality assurance which general practice will need to guarantee to retain its pivotal position in the UK health care system (see Figures 10 and 11).

David Colin-Thomé in Cheshire and Rhidian Morris in Devon are two others who have brought their local authority councellor experience formidably to bear in the creation of the National Association of Fundholding Practices (NAFP) to go alongside their continuing professional GP practice – and there are several others. (They are by no means all men either – Dr Jacky Hayden, GP and Regional Postgraduate Education Adviser in the North West NHS Region or Diane Plamping and Hilary Scott, Community Health Services leaders in South London, could just as easily be cited as renaissance figures.) Some are the new Regional Directors of Research and Development; perhaps in structural terms, given their access to major funding resources and position in the NHSE hierarchy, the office for clinicians that now offers the most obvious power and influence over future policy development. It is a far cry from the days, only a decade ago, when the (secondary care) College consultant bigwigs alone could command access to Downing Street.

These contemporary renaissance figures – Irvine, Pietroni, Carruthers, Hayden, Edwards and the rest – are all genuine friends to primary care. They are each excellent communicators. Legitimized by their alternative academic roles, they write prolifically and without inhibition.[2] They see and set the future agenda. By constantly positioning themselves formally and informally so that they can ensure their ideas are turned into tangible organizational processes and service outcomes, they have put together the platform for the next stage of NHS development. Their contribution has been the vital one in supplying the means by which the NHS can re-form itself.

NOTES

1   *The Dorset Story* is told in Carruthers I, Fillingham D *et al.* (1995) *Purchasing in the NHS: the story so far.* HSMC, University of Birmingham, pp 3–19.

2   Characteristic examples of the writings of the contemporary leaders of health services development described in this chapter are set out below. In the case of Sir Donald Irvine and David Colin-Thomé, in particular, the output qualifies as prolific.

   For the clearest statement of his vision for the future of the NHS, see Carruthers I (1994) Total fundholding in the mainstream of the NHS. *Primary Care Management* 4(3): 7–9.

   Brian Edwards' perspective on the development of the NHS and the importance of it becoming more responsive to ordinary people is well captured in the following two publications: Edwards B (1995) *The National Health Service: a manager's tale 1946–94.* Nuffield Provincial Hospitals Trust, London and NHSME (1992) *Local Voices: the views of local people in purchasing for health.* Department of Health, London.

   Sir Donald Irvine's most distinctive recent written contributions, often in partnership with his wife Sally, have been designed to extend the concept of quality and its application in primary care. They include Irvine D (1990) *Managing for Quality in General Practice.* King's Fund, London; Irvine D and Irvine S (1997) *Making Sense of Audit* (Second edn). Radcliffe Medical Press, Oxford; and Irvine D and Irvine S (1996) *The Practice of Quality.* Radcliffe Medical Press, Oxford.

   Happily the vision for primary care demonstrated by Patrick Pietroni in his practice, research and education programmes and writings is now brought together in Pietroni P and Pietroni C (eds) (1996) *Innovation in Community Care and Primary Health.* Churchill Livingstone, London.

   As Chairman of the National Association of Fundholding Practices (NAFP), Dr Morris has been able to use the monthly *Fundholding* magazine as a regular vehicle for his views. His perspective on the benefits of primary care-led purchasing are well set out in Morris R (1995) *Achievements of fundholders*, in Henry S and Pickersgill D (eds) (1995) *Making Sense of Fundholding*. Radcliffe Medical Press, Oxford.

Chapters on different aspects of the Castlefields Project at Runcorn in Cheshire have become a regular feature of contemporary collected essays. See, for example, Colin-Thomé D (1994) *Practice population commissioning*, in Peel V, Sheaffe R and Higgins J (eds) *Best Practice in Healthcare Commissioning*. Longman, Harlow; Colin-Thomé D (1995) *Future developments*, in Henry S and Pickersgill D (eds) *Making Sense of Fundholding*. Radcliffe Medical Press, Oxford; and Colin-Thomé D (1996) *The total fundholder*, in Meads G (ed.) *Future Options for General Practice*. Radcliffe Medical Press, Oxford.

7

Reformation *and* Enlightenment

'The hope of the world is still in dedicated minorities.'*

THE SUBJECTIVE REALITY OF THE MODERN NHS

By drawing on some of the most significant moments in history as the headings for the chapters in this book, I have sought to capture the way the NHS has felt to one participant observer during the 1990s. The moments selected have each been chosen deliberately as reference points for the tensions and pressures associated with the remarkable process of accelerated internal development which has taken place in the contemporary NHS. It has been an explosive experience, or rather range of experiences, each one colliding into another, leaving every individual with their own version of events, their own very different perceptions and understanding of the NHS itself. It has felt as though all history has been condensed into the space of a few short years.

This shift from objective to subjective reality was best captured

---

*Martin Luther King, the assassinated black American civil rights leader, on justice and freedom in *The Words of Martin Luther King: selected by his widow Loretta Scott King* (1984) Robson Books, London.

for me when I helped facilitate a three-day learning event on the impact of a primary care-led NHS, in November 1995.[1] The contemporary NHS, as the following account illustrates so vividly, presented itself as a contradiction in terms. On the one hand radical variations in perception emerged in respect of today's NHS relationships and how they affect its future policy development; while on the other the pervasive conservatism of the different players and their innate desire to stay together, both for and within the traditional structures of the NHS family, was plain to see. Their profound ambiguities were demonstrated most clearly by the group of FHSA/DHA/RHA members.

They were the last group of course participants to report and, according to popular stereotype, the least promising. Largely central appointees and female, the most senior in both status and age, their feedback at the regional learning event seemed likely to be the most conservative. Not that it would really matter; the material from the first four groups had been sufficiently stimulating. There had been more than enough for the facilitators to exploit over the remaining two days of the programme.

The Purchaser Chief Executives group had mapped the relationships of the reformed NHS on an imaginary dartboard covered with one-off 'hits'. Around the bulls-eye were stuck three pieces of paper bearing the titles 'Secretary of State', 'GPs', and 'HA Chief Executives' – of course! This triumvirate of power was surrounded by a bewildering mosaic of other paper patches and concentric circles, the wording on which was too hard to read, let alone understand, from any distance away. In short, it was chaos theory; the reformed NHS – too complex to communicate – with GPs and Ministers in exclusive control and top level general management mediating between them. The message was clear enough; only they were in a position to interpret what was really going on and hold the NHS together.

The Provider Representatives were a little less graphic. The 'electrical circuits' they drew contained pathetically few points and quickly looped back to the original socket; the NHS Trust itself. The Community Trust did have a 'terminal' with the Social Services Department but otherwise its circuit followed the same sparse lines as its Acute counterpart. Together it seemed they had lost contact with the external NHS. They did not really know what was happening in the wider world.

The Primary Care Team players felt very much the same, at least at practice management level. Their image of the reformed NHS was of a five-layer pyramid with the Government and NHS Executive at the top, providers and purchasers as the solid intervening layers and general practice the burgeoning bottom tier. There was only one problem with this expansion; the overall height of the pyramid was not changing. The pressure at the bottom was simply much heavier, getting closer and closer to bursting point, and those at the top of the pyramid remained out of sight and out of reach.

As described earlier in Chapter 1, a galaxy of stars, planets and constellations was the image of the fourth set of stakeholders; the service users and their representatives. Shooting stars and short-life meteorites briefly caught the eye: GP fundholders, health commissioners and purchasing strategies. It was, however, the Department of Health as the sun that dominated the skyline. While the former burnt out, this everlasting orb blazed ever more brightly, shedding light on all those that stayed within its rays. The users and carers were not sure that they should have been paired, but together they knew exactly to whom they should still relate in the reformed NHS. Over time the universe stays the same.

After four such vivid and varying illustrations of subjective reality in the reformed NHS of the 1990s, there seemed there could be little more to add when, unexpectedly, all those in the non-Executive member stakeholder group got up and came to the front of the room. They stood, Indian-file, in a line with one of their number set apart, calling the tune. At her instruction, the leader of the line spoke:

'It is the pre-primary care-led NHS and I am the Consultant, and I lead the NHS.'

'And I am a University and I follow the Consultant', said the next in line.

'Me, too', echoed the third person, an NHS Manager.

'And I am a GP and I am where I am used to being; stuck in the middle and unable to get out', said the next, facing the back of the manager who was facing the back of the University representative ahead of him. Their procession was an orderly, even spaced one.

Next in the row, after a gap, was the CHC complaining of neglect but still looking nevertheless in exactly the same direction as the others; and then finally, after a larger interval of time and space, came the Patient:

'I'm at the back and I cannot even see the front of the queue. That's where the Consultant is, isn't it? I thought he was meant to be looking after me.'

The member set apart from the line then spoke again announcing:

'I am the Regional Chair. It is now 1 April 1996. The primary care-led NHS is upon us.'

What happened next? Who moved in the column? Certainly not the Consultant who stayed at its head. The University representative remarked that she only changed course 'very slowly' and even the GP was reluctant to shift his stance until sharply reminded again that these were the days of the *primary care-led* NHS, which forced him to half-turn and face the CHC for the first time, with disturbing effect:

'I don't like this at all', said their representative. 'Now we are faced with all these local practices. There are far too many of them for us to cope with and most of them won't let us in. Even if they do, we cannot see what they are up to. It's not like ward rounds; the consulting room door is always shut.'

One person did make a 180-degree turn, the NHS Manager, as directed. But this did not last long. In a parting statement the RHA Chair proclaimed a centrally imposed eight per cent reduction in 'overheads'. The NHS Manager stepped aside, then so too did the RHA Chair herself. They were no longer on the map of the reformed NHS, leaving it as it was before, in the same order but only with wider gaps. They had both been made redundant. The Patient's concluding cry now was the same:

'I am still at the back and now nobody seems to know where we should be going. I liked the sound of a primary care-led NHS, but now, who is going to make it happen?'

CREATING A NEW ORTHODOXY FOR THE NHS

Reformation in history applies to the phases when the different, diverse strands of strategic development start finally to come together. A new orthodoxy is created, with roots in a past that long precedes the more immediate periods of upheaval; and with substantial popular support right across society. Witness the birth of the Lutheran and Anglican traditions – new churches in their time, belonging very much to their nation states and yet still claiming a direct line descendancy to the first Apostles.

So it can be now with an NHS about to reach its half century and enter a new millennium. The basic values remain the same, only the form changes. In the past clinical specialisms led the way defining professional and personal identities with management and organizations following in their wake. The new focus on care reverses this order and the development cycle (see Figure 12). The important thing for the NHS at the end of the present turbulent decade is that it should be true to both its history and its future.

This means that *choice* must be added to the list of original core values of a free, equal and comprehensive health service. It means re-forming its structure and processes around the changes at its bedrock, in gatekeeping general practice. Given its cost and clinical pressures, the NHS cannot continue sensibly to support and subsidise over 9000 small businesses and no modern public utility or service has anything like as many as one hundred local regulatory bodies. These figures apply, of course, to the present numbers of general practices and health authorities respectively. Reductions

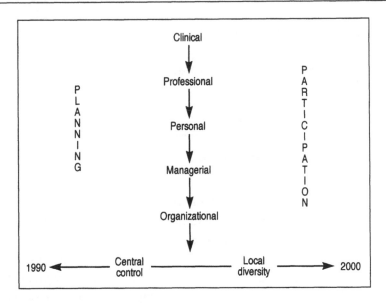

Figure 12: NHS development sequence.

of a third and a half are realistic expectations as the franchising of primary managed care organizations, combining purchasing and providing functions, becomes the norm (see Figure 4, p 17). The reformation of the NHS is now just about in sight, re-forming after the revolutionary years with their dark ages, in ways that are true to its previous history.

This means planning for the NHS as a whole within manageable geographic limits. It means ensuring sufficient local availability of specialist acute services. It means promoting the integration of health and social services in primary care.[2] These three statements in turn represent the re-visiting of the fundamental NHS developments of 1948, 1962 and 1974; of the establishment of regions, of hospital plans and health centres. By the year 2000 we will see added to these – as a result of including *choice* in NHS core values – provider trusts able to call fully upon both public and independent sector status and sources of support; just as, in fact, hospitals used to prior to 1945. Health care is a historic constant and its organization tends to turn full circle.

So too, many will hope, does NHS behaviour. Neither collaboration nor competition are without their moral pitfalls. Both are now

---

From GP to primary care partnerships requires:

- GPs respecting role of management and vice versa
- recognizing 'Good Health' has to equal 'Good Business'
- power sharing
- finding a common language
- listening

Figure 13: From GP to primary care partnerships.

legitimate vehicles for *development* which, applied to the contemporary health care system, now extends across a very broad range of approaches and styles. Both can be conducted with civility. As Figure 13 suggests, communication is the key. This checklist was drawn up by general practice and new health authority representatives working together on the crucial topic of 'Commissioning Primary Care Development' in an autumn HMG programme at City University. To each other's horror, after two days of the course, their lists of needs and resources hardly overlapped at all. So many meetings decline through misunderstanding, usually more accidental than by design. Contemporary NHS development, more than ever given its complexities, relies on checking out where others are coming from. Aspirations are usually exploratory and half-considered; language changes its meaning too often and, above all, every perspective today is decidedly partial.

FUTURE HOPES

For a while in the 1990s it has felt to participant observers of the NHS, like myself, as if developments in the UK health care system were somehow in defiance of the natural laws, upon which Thomas Hobbes based the words quoted at the beginning of Chapter 1. The world seemed to be like oceans without continents. At times and too often, amoral, aggressive, with few fixed points, the environment has been like a seascape of archipelagoes and islands with floating wrecks and patrolling gunboats in between. The reformation of the NHS offers a different prospect. The mainland is now visible on the horizon. It never went away. And it is the wood from the wrecks and the scrap metal from the frigates that can help us to form the bridges to take us back there. Reformation of the NHS is at hand; from which may even follow a further historical epoch: the Age of Enlightenment.

NOTES

1 This account is based on Meads G (1997) *Introduction* in Meads G, Huntington J, Key P *et al. The Unsupported Middle: future developments in a primary care-led NHS*. Radcliffe Medical Press, Oxford.

2 Examples of leading edge practice on the integration of health and social services in primary care within an overall framework for collaboration are contained in the Department of Health's newsletter for community care development programmes, entitled *Building Partnerships* (available from PO Box 235, Hayes, Middlesex, UB3 1HF) and Meads G (ed.) (1997) *Health and Social Services in Primary Care: an effective combination?* Churchill Livingstone, London.

Index

9 781857 752700